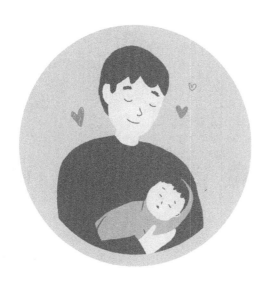

First-Time Dad

Journal

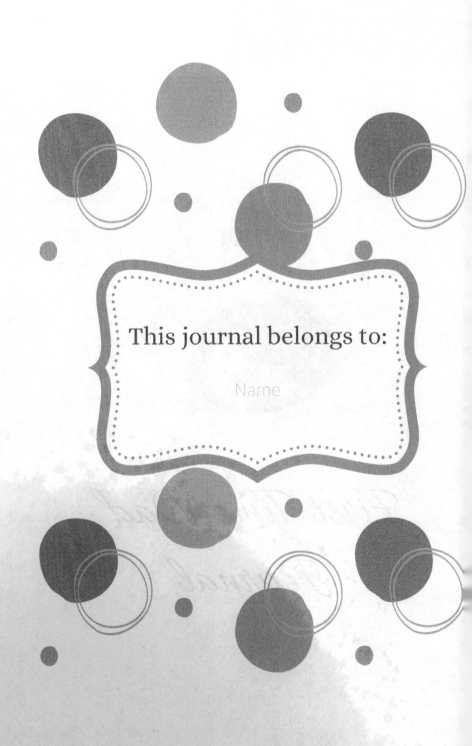

This journal belongs to:

Name

First-time dad journal   Date:

WE ARE HAVING A BABY!!

When I found out:

_____

_____

_____

_____

_____

_____

_____

_____

_____

_____

_____

_____

_____

_____

_____

_____

_____

_____

_____

_____

_____

First-time dad journal   Date:

How I found out:
_____
_____
_____
_____
_____
_____
_____
_____
_____
_____
_____
_____
_____
_____
_____
_____
_____
_____
_____
_____
_____
_____
_____
_____

First-time dad journal   Date:

Our feelings:
_____
_____
_____
_____
_____
_____
_____
_____
_____
_____
_____
_____
_____
_____
_____
_____
_____
_____
_____
_____
_____
_____
_____

Prenatal Appointment

Date:

Ultra Sound Picture Here!

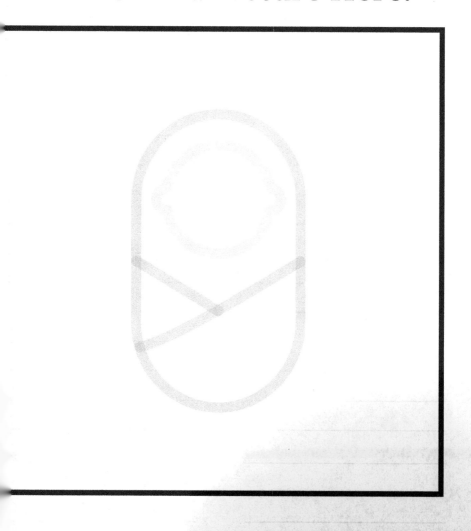

First-time dad journal   Date:

Boy Names ♂

Name: Suggested By:

_____   _____
_____   _____
_____   _____
_____   _____
_____   _____
_____   _____
_____   _____
_____   _____
_____   _____
_____   _____
_____   _____
_____   _____
_____   _____
_____   _____
_____   _____
_____   _____
_____   _____
_____   _____

Girl Names ♀

Name: Suggested By:

_____   _____

_____   _____

_____   _____

_____   _____

_____   _____

_____   _____

_____   _____

_____   _____

_____   _____

_____   _____

_____   _____

_____   _____

_____   _____

_____   _____

_____   _____

_____   _____

_____   _____

Date:

Mommy's Routine

First-time dad journal

Date:

_____

_____

_____

_____

_____

_____

_____

_____

_____

_____

_____

_____

_____

_____

_____

_____

_____

_____

_____

_____

_____

_____

_____

Baby Shower

Date: _____
Location: _____
Hosted by: _____

Gift	From	

first-time dad journal

Date:

Birth Plan!

_____
_____
_____
_____
_____
_____
_____
_____
_____
_____
_____
_____
_____
_____

First-time dad journal

Date:

_____

_____

_____

_____

_____

_____

_____

_____

_____

_____

_____

_____

_____

_____

_____

_____

_____

_____

_____

_____

_____

First-time dad journal

Date:

First-time dad journal

Highlights
of birth plan

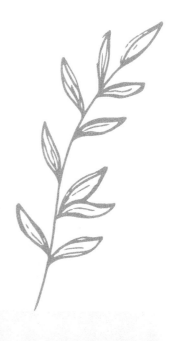

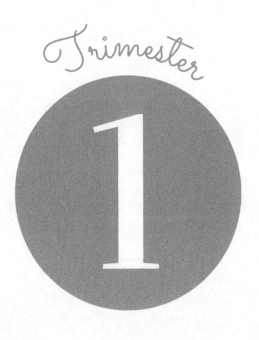

Date:

Week 1-4

_____
_____
_____
_____
_____
_____
_____
_____
_____
_____
_____
_____
_____
_____
_____
_____
_____
_____
_____
_____
_____
_____
_____
_____
_____

First-time dad journal

Date:

First-time dad journal

Date:

First-time dad journal

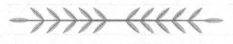

Highlights
of week 1-4

-c-c-c-c-c-

2

Week 5-8

First-time dad journal

Date:

irst-time dad journal   Date:

_____
_____
_____
_____
_____
_____
_____
_____
_____
_____
_____
_____
_____
_____
_____
_____
_____
_____
_____
_____
_____
_____

Highlights
of week 5-8

First-time dad journal

Date:

-c-c-c-c-c-

3

Week 9-13

First-time dad journal

Date:

_____

_____

_____

_____

_____

_____

_____

_____

_____

_____

_____

_____

_____

_____

_____

_____

_____

_____

_____

_____

_____

Date:

Appointment details: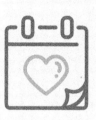

First-time dad journal

Date:

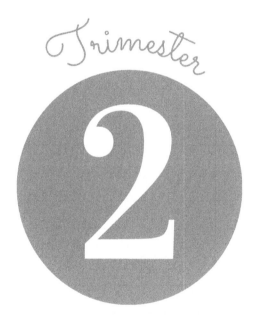

First-time dad journal

Date:

Week 14-17

First-time dad journal

Date:

First-time dad journal

Date:

Highlights
of week 14-17

5

Week 18-21

irst-time dad journal   Date:

_____

_____

_____

_____

_____

_____

_____

_____

_____

_____

_____

_____

_____

_____

_____

_____

_____

_____

_____

_____

_____

_____

_____

First-time dad journal

Date:

_____

_____

_____

_____

_____

_____

_____

_____

_____

_____

_____

_____

_____

_____

_____

_____

_____

_____

_____

_____

_____

_____

_____

Highlights
of week 18-21

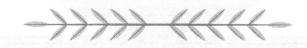

6

Week 22-26

First-time dad journal

Date:

_____

_____

_____

_____

_____

_____

_____

_____

_____

_____

_____

_____

_____

_____

_____

_____

_____

_____

_____

_____

_____

_____

_____

Appointment details:

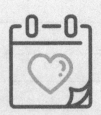

Highlights
of week 22-26

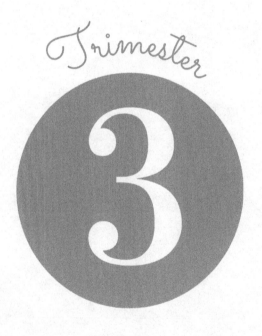

First-time dad journal

Date:

Week 27-30

First-time dad journal

Date:

First-time dad journal   Date:

_____

_____

_____

_____

_____

_____

_____

_____

_____

_____

_____

_____

_____

_____

_____

_____

_____

_____

_____

_____

_____

_____

_____

_____

_____

First-time dad journal

Highlights
of week 27-30

Date:

Week 31-35

First-time dad journal

Date:

First-time dad journal

Date:

_____

_____

_____

_____

_____

_____

_____

_____

_____

_____

_____

_____

_____

_____

_____

_____

_____

_____

_____

_____

_____

_____

_____

First-time dad journal

Highlights
of week 31-38

-C-C-C-C-C-

9

Week 36-40

First-time dad journal

Date:

Date:

Appointment details:

First-time dad journal

Date:

Highlights
of week 36-40

TIME TO MEET
YOU

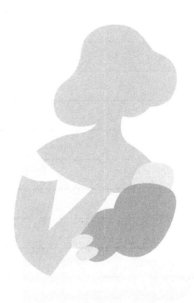

First-time dad journal

Date:

First-time dad journal   Date:

_____

_____

_____

_____

_____

_____

_____

_____

_____

_____

_____

_____

_____

_____

_____

_____

_____

_____

_____

_____

_____

_____

_____

First-time dad journal

Date:

_____

_____

_____

_____

_____

_____

_____

_____

_____

_____

_____

_____

_____

_____

_____

_____

_____

_____

_____

_____

_____

irst-time dad journal   Date:

_____
_____
_____
_____
_____
_____
_____
_____
_____
_____
_____
_____
_____
_____
_____
_____
_____
_____
_____
_____
_____
_____
_____
_____

Birth plan vs Reality

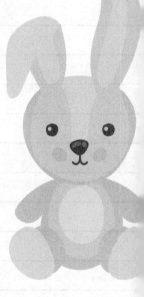

First-time dad journal

Date:

First-time dad journal

Date:

First-time dad journal   Date:

_____

_____

_____

_____

_____

_____

_____

_____

_____

_____

_____

_____

_____

_____

_____

_____

_____

_____

_____

_____

_____

_____

_____

_____

Labour & Delivery Story

First-time dad journal

Date:

First-time dad journal

Date:

First-time dad journal

Date:

First-time dad journal

Date:

Date:

YOUR
ARRIVAL

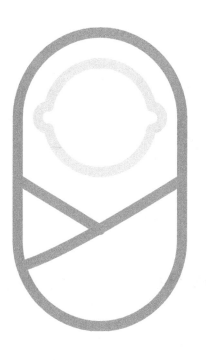

Date of Birth   _____

Time of Birth   _____

Weight   _____

Height   _____

Baby Picture

First-time dad journal

Date:

My First
THOUGHTS

_____
_____
_____
_____
_____
_____
_____
_____
_____
_____
_____
_____

First-time dad journal

Date:

Date:

First-time dad journal

Date:

Date:

Highlights
of thoughts

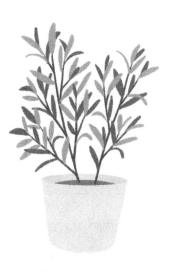

First-time dad journal

Date:

First-time dad journal

Date:

First-time dad journal

Date:

_____

_____

_____

_____

_____

_____

_____

_____

_____

_____

_____

_____

_____

_____

_____

_____

_____

_____

_____

_____

_____

_____

_____

_____

First-time dad journal

Date:

Date:

_____

_____

_____

_____

_____

_____

_____

_____

_____

_____

_____

_____

_____

_____

_____

_____

_____

_____

_____

_____

_____

_____

_____

All about You!!

First-time dad journal

Date:

First-time dad journal

Date:

Date:

Nicknames

First-time dad journal

Date:

---

rst-time dad journal   Date:

_____
_____
_____
_____
_____
_____
_____
_____
_____
_____
_____
_____
_____
_____
_____
_____
_____
_____
_____
_____
_____
_____
_____
_____

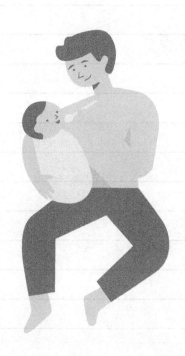

Picture with dad!

First-time dad journal

Date:

First-time dad journal

Date:

Highlights about you

first-time dad journal   Date:

_____
_____
_____
_____
_____
_____
_____
_____
_____
_____
_____
_____
_____
_____
_____
_____
_____
_____
_____
_____
_____
_____
_____
_____
_____

First-time dad journal

Date:

First-time dad journal

Date:

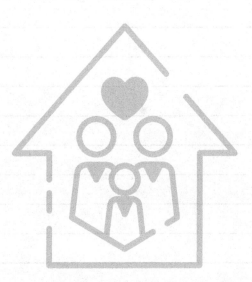

Family picture

Made in the USA
Monee, IL
10 October 2024

67592976R00056